KIDNEY DISEASE DIET COOKBOOK FOR SENIORS

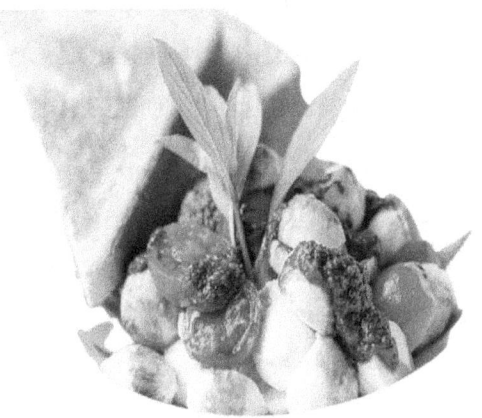

Delicious and Nutritious Recipes for Managing Kidney Health in Your Golden Years

Tina Feldman

Copyright © Tina Feldman 2024

All rights reserved. No part of this publication may be reproduced, distributed, or transmitted in any form or by any means, including photocopying, recording or other electronic or mechanical methods, without the prior written permission of the publisher, except in the case of brief quotations embodied in critical reviews and certain other non-commercial uses permitted by copyright law.

Table of Contents

INTRODUCTION 7

PART 1: Understanding Kidney Disease and the Importance of Diet for Seniors 9

   Importance of Diet for Seniors with Kidney Disease: 10

   Benefits of a Kidney-Friendly Diet 12

   Meal planning tips 14

   Tips for dining out with kidney diseases 17

   Food to Limit or Avoid 20

   Food to eat 23

PART 2: HEALTHY AND DELICIOUS RECIPES 26

BREAKFAST 26

   1. Veggie Omelette 26

   2. Overnight Oats with Berries 27

   3. Greek Yogurt Parfait 28

   4. Spinach and Feta Breakfast Wrap 29

   5. Cottage Cheese Pancakes 29

   6. Avocado Toast with Poached Egg 30

   7. Quinoa Breakfast Bowl 31

   8. Breakfast Smoothie Bowl 32

   9. Egg Muffins with Spinach and Turkey Bacon 33

10. Tofu Scramble with Vegetables 34

LUNCH 35

1. Grilled Chicken Salad with Citrus Dressing .. 35
2. Vegetable Stir-Fry with Tofu 36
3. Lentil Soup with Spinach 37
4. Turkey and Avocado Wrap 38
5. Quinoa and Black Bean Salad 39
6. Salmon Salad Sandwich 40
7. Eggplant and Tomato Pasta 41
8. Veggie Burger with Sweet Potato Fries 42
9. Chickpea Salad with Lemon Tahini Dressing 43
10. Tuna Salad Lettuce Wraps 44

DINNER 45

1. Baked Salmon with Lemon-Dill Sauce 45
2. Quinoa-Stuffed Bell Peppers 46
3. Chicken and Vegetable Stir-Fry 47
4. Lentil and Vegetable Soup 48
5. Turkey Meatballs with Marinara Sauce 49
6. Veggie-Packed Frittata 50
7. Shrimp and Vegetable Stir-Fry 51
8. Baked Chicken Breast with Herbs 52

9. Eggplant Parmesan 53

10. Tofu and Vegetable Curry 54

SMOOTHIES 55

1. Berry Blast Smoothie 55

2. Green Power Smoothie 56

3. Tropical Delight Smoothie 56

4. Creamy Peanut Butter Banana Smoothie 57

5. Creamy Coconut and Berry Smoothie 58

6. Peachy Green Smoothie 58

7. Mocha Almond Smoothie 59

8. Cherry Vanilla Smoothie 60

9. Pineapple Ginger Smoothie 61

10. Watermelon Mint Cooler Smoothie 61

SNACKS AND APPETIZER 63

1. Veggie Sticks with Hummus 63

2. Greek Yogurt with Berries 63

3. Cucumber Avocado Rolls 64

4. Apple Slices with Almond Butter 65

5. Rice Cake with Cottage Cheese and Tomato 66

6. Baked Sweet Potato Chips 66

7. Tuna Cucumber Bites 67

8. Edamame with Sea Salt 68

9. Bell Pepper Nachos 68

10. Cottage Cheese Stuffed Cherry Tomatoes. 69

BONUS 70

Shopping lists 70

CONCLUSION 77

INTRODUCTION

Welcome to "Nourishing Wellness: A Kidney Disease Diet Cookbook for Seniors." This cookbook is crafted with care and expertise to provide seniors with kidney disease a wealth of flavorful, satisfying, and nourishing recipes tailored to their specific dietary needs.

As we age, our bodies undergo various changes, and for many seniors, managing kidney health becomes a significant concern. Kidney disease, whether chronic or acute, requires careful attention to diet and nutrition. My goal with this cookbook is to empower seniors with kidney disease to make delicious and healthful choices every day, supporting their overall wellness and quality of life.

Within these pages, you'll find a diverse array of recipes thoughtfully designed to meet the dietary restrictions commonly associated with kidney disease. From breakfast to dinner, and everything in between, each recipe has been crafted to be low in sodium, potassium, and phosphorus, while still being rich in essential nutrients and flavor. We've also provided detailed nutritional information for each recipe, ensuring that seniors can easily track their intake and make informed choices.

But this cookbook is more than just a collection of recipes. It's a guide to navigating the challenges of kidney disease with confidence and creativity. In addition to delicious meal ideas, you'll find practical tips for grocery shopping, meal planning, dining out, and more. We believe that with the right knowledge and resources, seniors with kidney disease can continue to enjoy a varied and fulfilling diet that supports their health and well-being.

Whether you're a senior managing kidney disease yourself or a caregiver looking to provide nutritious meals for a loved one, "Nourishing Wellness" is here to inspire and support you on your journey to better health. Let's embark on this culinary adventure together, one delicious and kidney-friendly recipe at a time.

PART 1: Understanding Kidney Disease and the Importance of Diet for Seniors

Understanding kidney disease is crucial for seniors as they are more susceptible to its onset and progression due to the natural aging process. Kidneys play a vital role in filtering waste products and excess fluids from the blood, maintaining electrolyte balance, and regulating blood pressure. However, with age, the kidneys may lose some of their efficiency, making seniors more prone to kidney problems. It's important for seniors and their caregivers to grasp the fundamentals of kidney disease and the significance of diet in managing it.

Understanding Kidney Disease:
1. Types of Kidney Disease: There are various types of kidney diseases, but the two most common among seniors are chronic kidney disease (CKD) and acute kidney injury (AKI). CKD is a gradual loss of kidney function over time, while AKI is a sudden loss of kidney function often caused by an acute illness or injury.

2. Causes and Risk Factors: Chronic conditions such as diabetes, hypertension, and heart disease are significant risk factors for kidney disease. Other risk factors include aging, smoking, obesity, and a family history of kidney disease.

3. Symptoms: Symptoms of kidney disease may not be apparent in the early stages. However, as the disease progresses, symptoms such as fatigue, swelling in the legs, ankles, or feet, changes in urine output, difficulty concentrating, and muscle cramps may manifest.

4. Diagnosis and Treatment: Diagnosis typically involves blood tests, urine tests, imaging tests like ultrasounds, and kidney biopsies. Treatment aims to slow the progression of the disease, manage symptoms, and prevent complications. Depending on the severity, treatments may include medications, lifestyle changes, dialysis, or kidney transplantation.

Importance of Diet for Seniors with Kidney Disease:

1. Controlling Protein Intake: Seniors with kidney disease may need to limit their protein intake as excessive protein consumption can strain the kidneys. However, it's essential to consult a healthcare provider or dietitian to determine the appropriate amount of protein based on individual needs.

2. Managing Sodium Intake: Sodium can increase blood pressure and fluid retention, putting extra strain on the kidneys. Seniors should limit their sodium intake by avoiding processed foods, canned goods, and restaurant meals, and opting for fresh, whole foods instead.

3. Monitoring Fluid Intake: Seniors with kidney disease may need to monitor their fluid intake, especially if they have fluid retention or are on dialysis. Too much fluid can lead to swelling and high blood pressure, while too little can cause dehydration.

4. Watching Potassium and Phosphorus Levels: High levels of potassium and phosphorus in the blood can be harmful to individuals with kidney disease. Seniors should be mindful of consuming foods high in these minerals, such as bananas, oranges, tomatoes, dairy products, and processed foods.

5. Emphasizing Nutrient-rich Foods: A diet rich in fruits, vegetables, whole grains, and lean proteins can provide essential nutrients while supporting overall health. However, portion control and moderation are key, especially for foods high in potassium, phosphorus, and protein.

6. Consulting a Dietitian: Each individual's dietary needs may vary based on their stage of kidney disease, overall health, medications, and other factors. Therefore, seniors with kidney disease should work closely with a registered dietitian who can create a personalized meal plan tailored to their specific needs and preferences.

Benefits of a Kidney-Friendly Diet

A kidney-friendly diet is crucial for seniors with kidney disease as it helps manage the condition, prevent complications, and improve overall health and well-being. Creating a kidney disease diet cookbook specifically tailored for seniors can provide practical guidance and delicious recipes that support kidney health. Here's a detailed exploration of the benefits such a cookbook can offer:

1. Education and Awareness:
    - Understanding Nutritional Needs: The cookbook can educate seniors about the specific nutritional needs of individuals with kidney disease, including protein, sodium, potassium, and phosphorus restrictions.
    - Awareness of Kidney-Friendly Foods: Seniors will learn which foods are beneficial for kidney health and which ones should be limited or avoided to prevent further damage to the kidneys.

2. Variety and Enjoyment:
    - Diverse Recipe Collection: The cookbook can offer a diverse collection of recipes ranging from appetizers and main courses to snacks and desserts, ensuring seniors have plenty of options to choose from.
    - Delicious and Flavorful Meals: By incorporating herbs, spices, and other flavorful ingredients, the cookbook can help seniors enjoy tasty meals while adhering to their dietary restrictions.

3. Nutritional Support:
    - Balanced Meal Planning: The cookbook can provide guidance on how to plan balanced meals that meet the nutritional needs of seniors with kidney disease, including portion control and meal timing.
    - Focus on Nutrient-Rich Foods: Recipes can emphasize nutrient-rich ingredients such as fruits, vegetables, whole grains, and lean proteins to ensure seniors receive essential vitamins and minerals.

4. Health Management:
    - Blood Pressure Control: A kidney-friendly diet can help seniors manage their blood pressure by limiting sodium intake and incorporating potassium-rich foods like sweet potatoes, spinach, and bananas.
    - Fluid Balance: Recipes can include tips for managing fluid intake, such as choosing foods with lower water content and monitoring portion sizes of fluid-rich foods like soups and stews.

5. Practical Tips and Advice:
    - Meal Preparation Techniques: The cookbook can offer practical tips and techniques for modifying recipes to meet dietary restrictions, such as using herbs and spices instead of salt for flavoring.
    - Shopping and Meal Planning Tips: Seniors can benefit from guidance on how to read food labels, make healthier choices at the grocery

store, and plan meals ahead of time to support their kidney health.

Meal planning tips

Meal planning is essential for seniors with kidney disease to ensure they follow a kidney-friendly diet that supports their health and well-being. Creating a kidney disease diet cookbook for seniors can include meal planning tips tailored to their specific dietary needs and restrictions. Here's a detailed exploration of meal planning tips for such a cookbook:

1. Understanding Dietary Restrictions:
   - Consult with Healthcare Professionals: Seniors should consult with their healthcare team, including dietitians and nephrologists, to understand their specific dietary restrictions based on their stage of kidney disease, lab results, and overall health.
   - Learn about Key Nutrients: Understanding the importance of limiting sodium, potassium, phosphorus, and protein intake can help seniors make informed decisions when planning their meals.
2. Building Balanced Meals:
   - Incorporate Variety: Encourage seniors to include a variety of foods from all food groups, such as fruits, vegetables, grains, lean proteins, and healthy fats, to ensure they receive a wide range of nutrients.
   - Focus on Portion Control: Emphasize the importance of portion control to avoid

overconsumption of nutrients that need to be limited, such as protein, sodium, and potassium.

3. Selecting Kidney-Friendly Foods:
   - Choose Low-Sodium Options: Opt for fresh or frozen fruits and vegetables, unsalted nuts and seeds, and low-sodium canned goods to reduce sodium intake.
   - Limit Potassium-Rich Foods: Encourage seniors to consume moderate amounts of potassium-rich foods such as bananas, oranges, and potatoes, and choose lower potassium alternatives when possible.
   - Monitor Phosphorus Intake: Select foods with lower phosphorus content, such as white bread, rice, and pasta, and limit high-phosphorus foods like dairy products, nuts, and seeds.

4. Meal Preparation Techniques:
   - Use Herbs and Spices: Encourage seniors to flavor their meals with herbs, spices, vinegar, lemon juice, and other low-sodium seasonings instead of salt to enhance taste without increasing sodium intake.
   - Experiment with Cooking Methods: Explore different cooking methods such as grilling, baking, steaming, and sautéing to add variety to meals while keeping them kidney-friendly.

5. Planning Ahead:

- Create a Weekly Meal Plan: Help seniors plan their meals for the week by selecting recipes that meet their dietary needs, considering leftovers and batch cooking to save time and effort.
- Make a Grocery List: Assist seniors in creating a grocery list based on their meal plan to ensure they have all the necessary ingredients on hand and avoid purchasing foods that may be harmful to their kidneys.

6. Stay Hydrated:
   - Monitor Fluid Intake: Encourage seniors to monitor their fluid intake and adjust it based on their individual needs, considering factors such as urine output, thirst, and activity level.
   - Choose Hydrating Foods: Incorporate hydrating foods such as cucumbers, watermelon, and lettuce into meals to help seniors maintain adequate hydration without exceeding fluid restrictions.

7. Seek Support and Resources:
   - Join Support Groups: Encourage seniors to join support groups or online communities for individuals with kidney disease to connect with others facing similar challenges, share experiences, and exchange meal ideas and recipes.
   - Consult with Dietitians: Recommend seniors to consult with a registered dietitian who specializes in kidney disease to receive

personalized meal planning guidance and support.

Tips for dining out with kidney diseases

Dining out can present challenges for seniors with kidney disease, as restaurant meals often contain high amounts of sodium, potassium, and phosphorus, which need to be limited to manage the condition effectively. However, with some careful planning and mindful choices, seniors can still enjoy dining out while adhering to their dietary restrictions. Here are some detailed tips for dining out with kidney disease:

1. Research Restaurants in Advance:
    - Choose Kidney-Friendly Restaurants: Look for restaurants that offer options suitable for a kidney-friendly diet, such as those that focus on fresh, whole foods and offer customizable meals.
    - Check Online Menus: Many restaurants now have their menus available online, allowing seniors to review options beforehand and identify dishes that align with their dietary restrictions.

2. Communicate with Restaurant Staff:
    - Inform Waitstaff about Dietary Needs: Upon arrival at the restaurant, inform the waiter or waitress about any dietary restrictions related to kidney disease, such as limiting sodium, potassium, and phosphorus.

- Ask for Modifications: Don't hesitate to ask if certain ingredients can be omitted or substituted to make a dish more kidney-friendly. Most restaurants are willing to accommodate special requests.

3. Make Smart Menu Choices:
   - Opt for Simple Preparations: Choose dishes that are prepared simply, such as grilled, baked, or steamed options, as they are likely to contain fewer added salts and seasonings.
   - Select Lean Proteins: Choose lean protein sources such as grilled chicken, fish, or tofu, and ask for sauces and dressings on the side to control sodium intake.

4. Be Mindful of Portion Sizes:
   - Share Entrées or Request Half Portions: Restaurant portion sizes are often larger than necessary, so consider sharing an entrée with a dining companion or requesting a half portion to avoid overeating.
   - Take Leftovers Home: If the portion size is still too large, don't hesitate to ask for a takeout container to bring leftovers home for another meal.

5. Watch Sodium Intake:
   - Request No Added Salt: Ask the restaurant to prepare your meal without added salt, and be cautious of foods that are typically high in sodium, such as soups, sauces, and processed meats.

- Avoid Condiments and Sauces: Limit the use of condiments like ketchup, soy sauce, and barbecue sauce, as they can be high in sodium. Instead, flavor your meal with lemon juice, herbs, or vinegar.

6. Monitor Potassium and Phosphorus:
    - Choose Low-Potassium Options: Select foods that are lower in potassium, such as rice, pasta, and steamed vegetables, and avoid high-potassium items like tomatoes, potatoes, and bananas.
    - Limit Phosphorus-Rich Foods: Be mindful of foods high in phosphorus, such as dairy products, nuts, and seeds, and choose alternatives with lower phosphorus content.

7. Stay Hydrated:
    - Choose Beverages Wisely: Opt for water, unsweetened tea, or other low-calorie, low-sodium beverages to stay hydrated without consuming excess fluids.
    - Limit Alcohol: If you choose to drink alcohol, do so in moderation, as it can dehydrate the body and interfere with medication.

8. Listen to Your Body:
Pay Attention to How You Feel: Be mindful of how certain foods affect your body and adjust your choices accordingly. If you experience symptoms like swelling or increased thirst, consider modifying your diet accordingly.

Food to Limit or Avoid

A kidney disease diet cookbook for seniors should include comprehensive guidance on foods to limit or avoid to support kidney health and manage the condition effectively. Seniors with kidney disease need to be mindful of their intake of certain nutrients, including sodium, potassium, phosphorus, and protein, as excessive amounts can exacerbate kidney damage and lead to complications. Here's a detailed exploration of foods to limit or avoid:

1. High-Sodium Foods:
    - Processed Meats: Deli meats, bacon, sausage, and hot dogs are high in sodium and should be limited or avoided.
    - Canned Foods: Canned soups, vegetables, and beans often contain added salt for preservation. Opt for low-sodium or no-salt-added varieties.
    - Packaged Snacks: Chips, pretzels, crackers, and other packaged snacks are typically high in sodium. Choose unsalted or low-sodium alternatives.
    - Condiments and Sauces: Soy sauce, ketchup, barbecue sauce, and salad dressings are often loaded with sodium. Look for low-sodium versions or use herbs and spices for flavoring instead.

2. High-Potassium Foods:
    - Bananas: Bananas are rich in potassium and should be limited or avoided by seniors with kidney disease.

- Oranges and Orange Juice: Oranges and orange juice are high in potassium. Consider consuming smaller portions or choosing lower-potassium fruits such as apples or berries.
- Tomatoes: Tomatoes and tomato products like sauces and soups are high in potassium. Opt for lower-potassium alternatives like bell peppers or cucumbers.
- Potatoes: Potatoes, including white, sweet, and red varieties, are high in potassium. Choose smaller portions and consider leaching or soaking them to reduce potassium content before cooking.

3. High-Phosphorus Foods:
   - Dairy Products: Milk, cheese, yogurt, and other dairy products are rich in phosphorus and should be consumed in moderation. Choose lower-phosphorus alternatives such as almond milk or nondairy cheese.
   - Nuts and Seeds: Almonds, peanuts, sunflower seeds, and other nuts and seeds are high in phosphorus. Limit portion sizes or choose lower-phosphorus options like rice cakes or air-popped popcorn.
   - Whole Grains: Whole grains such as whole wheat, brown rice, and quinoa contain more phosphorus than refined grains. Opt for smaller portions or choose refined grain alternatives.

4. High-Protein Foods:

- Red Meat: Beef, pork, and lamb are high in protein and should be limited, especially for seniors with advanced kidney disease. Choose lean cuts and smaller portions.
- Processed Meats: In addition to being high in sodium, processed meats like bacon, sausage, and deli meats are also high in protein. Choose lower-protein alternatives or limit portion sizes.
- Eggs: Eggs are a significant source of protein and phosphorus. Limit egg consumption to a few times per week or consider using only egg whites.

5. Fluid-Restricted Foods:
    - High-Water Content Fruits and Vegetables: Seniors with fluid restrictions may need to limit their intake of high-water content fruits and vegetables such as watermelon, cucumbers, and celery.
    - Soups and Broths: Soups, broths, and other liquid-based foods can contribute to fluid intake. Choose lower-sodium and lower-fluid alternatives or limit portion sizes.

6. Miscellaneous:
    - Artificial Sweeteners: Some artificial sweeteners may contain phosphorus additives. Check labels carefully or opt for natural sweeteners like stevia.
    - Alcohol: Alcohol can affect kidney function and may interact with medications. Limit alcohol

consumption or avoid it altogether, especially if you have advanced kidney disease.

Food to eat

A kidney disease diet cookbook for seniors should feature a variety of delicious and nutritious recipes that support kidney health and align with dietary restrictions. Incorporating foods that are low in sodium, potassium, phosphorus, and protein can help seniors manage their condition effectively and improve overall well-being. Here's a detailed exploration of foods to include in a kidney disease diet cookbook for seniors:

1. Low-Sodium Foods:
    - Fresh Fruits and Vegetables: Choose a variety of colorful fruits and vegetables such as apples, berries, grapes, broccoli, carrots, and leafy greens. These foods are naturally low in sodium and rich in essential vitamins and minerals.
    - Whole Grains: Opt for whole grains such as brown rice, quinoa, barley, and oats, which are lower in sodium compared to processed grains. Use whole grains as the base for salads, soups, and side dishes.
    - Lean Proteins: Select lean protein sources such as skinless poultry, fish, tofu, and legumes. These options are lower in sodium and saturated fat compared to red meat and processed meats.

2. Low-Potassium Foods:
   - Apples and Berries: Enjoy apples, berries, cherries, and grapes as delicious and kidney-friendly snacks or toppings for oatmeal and yogurt.
   - Cruciferous Vegetables: Include vegetables like cauliflower, cabbage, and Brussels sprouts in salads, stir-fries, and roasted vegetable dishes. These vegetables are low in potassium and high in fiber.
   - White Bread and Pasta: Choose white bread, pasta, and rice over whole grain varieties, as they contain less potassium. Use these options as part of balanced meals with lean protein and vegetables.

3. Low-Phosphorus Foods:
   - Egg Whites: Incorporate egg whites into omelets, scrambles, and baked goods as a lower-phosphorus alternative to whole eggs. Egg whites are rich in protein and low in phosphorus.
   - Cooked Vegetables: Enjoy a variety of cooked vegetables such as green beans, asparagus, zucchini, and peppers. Boiling or steaming vegetables can help reduce phosphorus content.
   - Non-Dairy Milk Alternatives: Choose non-dairy milk alternatives like almond milk, rice milk, or coconut milk that are lower in phosphorus compared to cow's milk.

4. Low-Protein Foods:
   - Plant-Based Proteins: Incorporate plant-based protein sources such as beans, lentils, tofu, and edamame into meals. These options are lower in protein compared to animal-based proteins and provide essential nutrients and fiber.
   - Grains and Starches: Include grains and starches such as rice, pasta, bread, and cereals in meals to complement plant-based proteins and add variety to the diet.
   - Vegetable-Based Soups: Prepare homemade vegetable-based soups using low-sodium broth, a variety of vegetables, and herbs and spices for flavor. Vegetable soups can be filling and nutritious while being lower in protein.

5. Fluid-Restricted Foods:
   - Portion-Controlled Fruits: Enjoy fruits in moderation, choosing options with lower water content such as apples, berries, and cherries. Portion control is essential for seniors with fluid restrictions.
   - Cooked Grains: Cook grains such as rice, quinoa, and couscous with measured amounts of water to control fluid intake. Use cooked grains as a base for salads, stir-fries, and pilafs.

6. Miscellaneous:
   - Healthy Fats: Incorporate healthy fats from sources such as avocados, nuts, seeds, and olive oil into meals and snacks. These fats provide

essential nutrients and add flavor and texture to dishes.
- Herbs and Spices: Use herbs, spices, vinegar, lemon juice, and citrus zest to flavor meals without adding salt or sodium-containing seasonings.

PART 2: HEALTHY AND DELICIOUS RECIPES

BREAKFAST

1. Veggie Omelette

Ingredients:
1. 2 large eggs
2. 1/4 cup diced bell peppers
3. 1/4 cup diced onions
4. 1/4 cup diced tomatoes
5. 1 tablespoon chopped fresh parsley
6. Cooking spray
7. Salt and pepper to taste (optional)

Preparation:
- In a bowl, whisk together eggs until well beaten.
- Heat a non-stick skillet over medium heat and coat with cooking spray.
- Pour beaten eggs into the skillet and swirl to coat the bottom evenly.

- Sprinkle diced vegetables and parsley over one half of the omelette.
- Cook until the edges start to set, then fold the other half over the filling.
- Cook for another 1-2 minutes until the omelette is cooked through.
- Season with salt and pepper if desired.

Nutritional Information (per serving):
- Sodium: 150mg
- Potassium: 190mg
- Phosphorus: 90mg
- Protein: 12g
- Calories: 150

2. Overnight Oats with Berries

Ingredients:
1. 1/2 cup rolled oats
2. 1/2 cup unsweetened almond milk
3. 1/4 cup fresh berries (such as blueberries or strawberries)
4. 1 tablespoon chia seeds
5. 1 tablespoon chopped almonds (optional)
6. 1 teaspoon honey (optional)

Preparation:
- In a mason jar or bowl, combine rolled oats and almond milk.
- Stir in chia seeds and chopped almonds if using.

- Cover and refrigerate overnight.
- In the morning, top with fresh berries and drizzle with honey if desired.

Nutritional Information (per serving):
- Sodium: 50mg
- Potassium: 140mg
- Phosphorus: 70mg
- Protein: 6g
- Calories: 200

3. Greek Yogurt Parfait

Ingredients:
1. 1/2 cup plain Greek yogurt
2. 1/4 cup granola (low-sodium and low-phosphorus)
3. 1/4 cup diced mango
4. 1 tablespoon sliced almonds
5. 1 teaspoon honey (optional)

Preparation:
- In a glass or bowl, layer Greek yogurt, granola, diced mango, and sliced almonds.
- Drizzle with honey if desired.

Nutritional Information (per serving):
- Sodium: 70mg
- Potassium: 180mg
- Phosphorus: 100mg
- Protein: 12g
- Calories: 220

4. Spinach and Feta Breakfast Wrap

Ingredients:
1. 1 whole wheat tortilla
2. 2 large eggs, scrambled
3. 1/4 cup cooked spinach
4. 2 tablespoons crumbled feta cheese
5. Salt and pepper to taste (optional)

Preparation:
- Warm the tortilla in a skillet or microwave.
- Fill the tortilla with scrambled eggs, cooked spinach, and crumbled feta cheese.
- Season with salt and pepper if desired.
- Roll up the tortilla to form a wrap.

Nutritional Information (per serving):
- Sodium: 220mg
- Potassium: 190mg
- Phosphorus: 130mg
- Protein: 14g
- Calories: 250

5. Cottage Cheese Pancakes

Ingredients:
1. 1/2 cup low-fat cottage cheese
2. 2 large eggs
3. 2 tablespoons oat flour
4. 1/2 teaspoon baking powder
5. 1/4 teaspoon vanilla extract
6. Cooking spray

Preparation:
- In a blender, combine cottage cheese, eggs, oat flour, baking powder, and vanilla extract. Blend until smooth.
- Heat a non-stick skillet over medium heat and coat with cooking spray.
- Pour small portions of the batter onto the skillet to form pancakes.
- Cook for 2-3 minutes on each side until golden brown.
- Serve with fresh fruit or a drizzle of honey if desired.

Nutritional Information (per serving):
- Sodium: 180mg
- Potassium: 200mg
- Phosphorus: 120mg
- Protein: 16g
- Calories: 230

6. Avocado Toast with Poached Egg

Ingredients:
1. 1 slice whole grain bread, toasted
2. 1/4 ripe avocado, mashed
3. 1 large egg, poached
4. Salt and pepper to taste (optional)
5. Chopped chives or parsley for garnish (optional)

Preparation:
- Spread mashed avocado onto the toasted bread.
- Top with a poached egg.
- Season with salt and pepper if desired.
- Garnish with chopped chives or parsley if desired.

Nutritional Information (per serving):
- Sodium: 100mg
- Potassium: 200mg
- Phosphorus: 150mg
- Protein: 12g
- Calories: 220

7. Quinoa Breakfast Bowl

Ingredients:
1. 1/2 cup cooked quinoa
2. 1/4 cup sliced strawberries
3. 1/4 cup diced pineapple
4. 2 tablespoons unsweetened coconut flakes
5. 1 tablespoon chopped almonds
6. 1 tablespoon honey (optional)

Preparation:
- In a bowl, layer cooked quinoa, sliced strawberries, diced pineapple, coconut flakes, and chopped almonds.
- Drizzle with honey if desired.

Nutritional Information (per serving):
- Sodium: 20mg

- Potassium: 180mg
- Phosphorus: 100mg
- Protein: 6g
- Calories: 220

8. Breakfast Smoothie Bowl

Ingredients:
- 1/2 cup unsweetened almond milk
- 1/2 frozen banana
- 1/2 cup frozen berries (such as blueberries or raspberries)
- 1/4 cup spinach leaves
- 1 tablespoon chia seeds
- 1 tablespoon unsweetened coconut flakes

Preparation:
1. In a blender, combine almond milk, frozen banana, frozen berries, spinach leaves, and chia seeds. Blend until smooth.
2. Pour the smoothie into a bowl and top with unsweetened coconut flakes.

Nutritional Information (per serving):
- Sodium: 50mg
- Potassium: 230mg
- Phosphorus: 80mg
- Protein: 5g
- Calories: 180

9. Egg Muffins with Spinach and Turkey Bacon

Ingredients:
1. 4 large eggs
2. 1/4 cup chopped spinach
3. 2 slices turkey bacon, cooked and crumbled
4. Salt and pepper to taste (optional)

Preparation:
- Preheat the oven to 350°F (175°C) and lightly grease a muffin tin.
- In a bowl, whisk together eggs until well beaten.
- Stir in chopped spinach and crumbled turkey bacon.
- Season with salt and pepper if desired.
- Divide the egg mixture evenly among the muffin cups.
- Bake for 15-20 minutes until the egg muffins are set and lightly golden.
- Allow to cool slightly before serving.

Nutritional Information (per serving, 2 egg muffins):
- Sodium: 220mg
- Potassium: 180mg
- Phosphorus: 100mg
- Protein: 14g
- Calories: 220

10. Tofu Scramble with Vegetables

Ingredients:
1. 1/2 cup extra-firm tofu, crumbled
2. 1/4 cup diced bell peppers
3. 1/4 cup diced onions
4. 1/4 cup diced tomatoes
5. 1/4 cup chopped spinach
6. 1/2 teaspoon turmeric powder
7. Salt and pepper to taste (optional)

Preparation:
- Heat a non-stick skillet over medium heat and add crumbled tofu.
- Cook for 2-3 minutes until tofu starts to brown.
- Add diced vegetables and turmeric powder to the skillet.
- Cook for another 3-4 minutes until vegetables are tender.
- Season with salt and pepper if desired.

Nutritional Information (per serving):
- Sodium: 130mg
- Potassium: 180mg
- Phosphorus: 90mg
- Protein: 10g
- Calories: 180

LUNCH

1. Grilled Chicken Salad with Citrus Dressing

Ingredients:
1. 4 oz grilled chicken breast, sliced
2. 2 cups mixed salad greens
3. 1/4 cup sliced cucumbers
4. 1/4 cup cherry tomatoes, halved
5. 1/4 cup mandarin orange segments
6. 1 tablespoon chopped walnuts (optional)
7. 2 tablespoons citrus vinaigrette dressing (low-sodium)

Preparation:
- Arrange mixed salad greens on a plate.
- Top with sliced grilled chicken, cucumbers, cherry tomatoes, and mandarin orange segments.
- Sprinkle chopped walnuts over the salad if desired.
- Drizzle with citrus vinaigrette dressing before serving.

Nutritional Information (per serving):
- Sodium: 150mg
- Potassium: 300mg
- Phosphorus: 150mg
- Protein: 25g
- Calories: 250

2. Vegetable Stir-Fry with Tofu

Ingredients:
1. 1/2 cup extra-firm tofu, cubed
2. 1 cup mixed stir-fry vegetables (such as bell peppers, broccoli, and snap peas)
3. 1 tablespoon low-sodium soy sauce
4. 1/2 tablespoon sesame oil
5. 1/4 teaspoon minced garlic
6. Cooked brown rice (optional, for serving)

Preparation:
- Heat sesame oil in a skillet over medium heat.
- Add minced garlic and cubed tofu to the skillet and cook until tofu is lightly browned.
- Add mixed stir-fry vegetables and cook until tender-crisp.
- Stir in low-sodium soy sauce and cook for an additional minute.
- Serve over cooked brown rice if desired.

Nutritional Information (per serving, without rice):
- Sodium: 120mg
- Potassium: 250mg
- Phosphorus: 100mg
- Protein: 15g
- Calories: 180

3. Lentil Soup with Spinach

Ingredients:
1. 1/2 cup dried green lentils, rinsed
2. 2 cups low-sodium vegetable broth
3. 1 cup chopped spinach
4. 1/4 cup diced carrots
5. 1/4 cup diced celery
6. 1/4 cup diced onions
7. 1/4 teaspoon ground cumin
8. Salt and pepper to taste (optional)

Preparation:
- In a large pot, combine dried lentils and vegetable broth.
- Bring to a boil, then reduce heat and simmer for 20-25 minutes until lentils are tender.
- Add chopped spinach, diced carrots, celery, onions, and ground cumin to the pot.
- Continue to simmer for an additional 10 minutes until vegetables are cooked through.
- Season with salt and pepper if desired before serving.

Nutritional Information (per serving):
- Sodium: 150mg
- Potassium: 300mg
- Phosphorus: 200mg
- Protein: 10g
- Calories: 200

4. Turkey and Avocado Wrap

Ingredients:
1. 1 whole wheat tortilla
2. 2 oz low-sodium deli turkey breast slices
3. 1/4 ripe avocado, sliced
4. 1/4 cup shredded lettuce
5. 1 tablespoon hummus (low-sodium)
6. 1 tablespoon diced tomatoes

Preparation:
- Lay the whole wheat tortilla flat and spread hummus evenly over the surface.
- Layer low-sodium deli turkey breast slices, sliced avocado, shredded lettuce, and diced tomatoes on top of the tortilla.
- Roll up the tortilla tightly to form a wrap.
- Slice the wrap in half before serving.

Nutritional Information (per serving):
- Sodium: 200mg
- Potassium: 220mg
- Phosphorus: 150mg
- Protein: 15g
- Calories: 220

5. Quinoa and Black Bean Salad

Ingredients:
1. 1/2 cup cooked quinoa
2. 1/4 cup canned black beans, rinsed and drained
3. 1/4 cup diced bell peppers
4. 1/4 cup diced tomatoes
5. 1/4 cup diced cucumbers
6. 2 tablespoons chopped cilantro
7. 1 tablespoon lime juice
8. 1 teaspoon olive oil
9. Salt and pepper to taste (optional)

Preparation:
- In a bowl, combine cooked quinoa, black beans, diced bell peppers, tomatoes, cucumbers, and chopped cilantro.
- Drizzle with lime juice and olive oil.
- Season with salt and pepper if desired.
- Toss gently to combine before serving.

Nutritional Information (per serving):
- Sodium: 120mg
- Potassium: 200mg
- Phosphorus: 100mg
- Protein: 8g
- Calories: 180

6. Salmon Salad Sandwich

Ingredients:
1. 2 oz canned salmon, drained and flaked
2. 1 tablespoon plain Greek yogurt
3. 1 tablespoon diced celery
4. 1 tablespoon diced red onion
5. 1 teaspoon lemon juice
6. Salt and pepper to taste (optional)
7. 2 slices whole grain bread

Preparation:
- In a bowl, combine flaked salmon, Greek yogurt, diced celery, diced red onion, and lemon juice.
- Season with salt and pepper if desired.
- Spread the salmon mixture onto one slice of whole grain bread.
- Top with the second slice of bread to form a sandwich.

Nutritional Information (per serving):
- Sodium: 180mg
- Potassium: 250mg
- Phosphorus: 180mg
- Protein: 15g
- Calories: 230

7. Eggplant and Tomato Pasta

Ingredients:
1. 1/2 cup whole wheat pasta, cooked
2. 1/2 cup diced eggplant
3. 1/4 cup diced tomatoes
4. 1/4 cup chopped spinach
5. 1/4 cup low-sodium marinara sauce
6. 1 tablespoon grated Parmesan cheese (optional)

Preparation:
- In a skillet, sauté diced eggplant until softened.
- Add diced tomatoes and chopped spinach to the skillet and cook until vegetables are tender.
- Stir in cooked whole wheat pasta and low-sodium marinara sauce.
- Cook for an additional 2-3 minutes until heated through.
- Serve hot, sprinkled with grated Parmesan cheese if desired.

Nutritional Information (per serving):
- Sodium: 150mg
- Potassium: 200mg
- Phosphorus: 100mg
- Protein: 8g
- Calories: 180

8. Veggie Burger with Sweet Potato Fries

Ingredients:
1. 1 veggie burger patty (low-sodium and low-phosphorus)
2. 1 whole grain burger bun
3. 1/2 cup baked sweet potato fries
4. Lettuce, tomato slices, and onion slices for topping (optional)

Preparation:
- Cook the veggie burger patty according to package instructions.
- Toast the whole grain burger bun until lightly browned.
- Assemble the burger by placing the cooked veggie burger patty on the bottom bun.
- Top with lettuce, tomato slices, and onion slices if desired.
- Serve with baked sweet potato fries on the side.

Nutritional Information (per serving):
- Sodium: 200mg
- Potassium: 250mg
- Phosphorus: 150mg
- Protein: 10g
- Calories: 220

9. Chickpea Salad with Lemon Tahini Dressing

Ingredients:
1. 1/2 cup canned chickpeas, rinsed and drained
2. 1/4 cup diced cucumbers
3. 1/4 cup diced tomatoes
4. 1/4 cup diced bell peppers
5. 2 tablespoons chopped parsley
6. 1 tablespoon lemon juice
7. 1 tablespoon tahini
8. Salt and pepper to taste (optional)

Preparation:
- In a bowl, combine chickpeas, diced cucumbers, tomatoes, bell peppers, and chopped parsley.
- In a small bowl, whisk together lemon juice and tahini to make the dressing.
- Drizzle the dressing over the chickpea salad and toss to coat.
- Season with salt and pepper if desired before serving.

Nutritional Information (per serving):
- Sodium: 150mg
- Potassium: 200mg
- Phosphorus: 100mg
- Protein: 8g
- Calories: 180

10. Tuna Salad Lettuce Wraps

Ingredients:
1. 2 oz canned tuna in water, drained
2. 1 tablespoon plain Greek yogurt
3. 1 tablespoon diced celery
4. 1 tablespoon diced red onion
5. 1 teaspoon Dijon mustard
6. Salt and pepper to taste (optional)
7. 4 large lettuce leaves

Preparation:
- In a bowl, combine canned tuna, Greek yogurt, diced celery, diced red onion, and Dijon mustard.
- Season with salt and pepper if desired.
- Spoon the tuna salad mixture onto lettuce leaves.
- Roll up the lettuce leaves to form wraps.

Nutritional Information (per serving, 2 lettuce wraps):
- Sodium: 200mg
- Potassium: 250mg
- Phosphorus: 180mg
- Protein: 20g
- Calories: 220

DINNER

1. Baked Salmon with Lemon-Dill Sauce

Ingredients:
1. 4 oz salmon fillet
2. 1 tablespoon lemon juice
3. 1/2 teaspoon dried dill
4. Salt and pepper to taste (optional)

Preparation:
- Preheat the oven to 400°F (200°C).
- Place the salmon fillet on a baking sheet lined with parchment paper.
- Drizzle lemon juice over the salmon and sprinkle with dried dill.
- Season with salt and pepper if desired.
- Bake for 12-15 minutes until the salmon is cooked through and flakes easily with a fork.
- Serve hot with a side of steamed vegetables.

Nutritional Information (per serving):
- Sodium: 80mg
- Potassium: 300mg
- Phosphorus: 200mg
- Protein: 25g
- Calories: 250

2. Quinoa-Stuffed Bell Peppers

Ingredients:
1. 2 large bell peppers, halved and seeded
2. 1/2 cup cooked quinoa
3. 1/4 cup black beans, rinsed and drained
4. 1/4 cup diced tomatoes
5. 1/4 cup diced onions
6. 1/4 cup chopped spinach
7. 1/4 teaspoon ground cumin
8. Salt and pepper to taste (optional)

Preparation:
- Preheat the oven to 375°F (190°C).
- In a bowl, combine cooked quinoa, black beans, diced tomatoes, onions, chopped spinach, ground cumin, salt, and pepper.
- Stuff the halved bell peppers with the quinoa mixture.
- Place the stuffed bell peppers in a baking dish and cover with foil.
- Bake for 25-30 minutes until the peppers are tender.
- Serve hot as a main dish.

Nutritional Information (per serving):
- Sodium: 120mg
- Potassium: 250mg
- Phosphorus: 150mg
- Protein: 10g
- Calories: 200

3. Chicken and Vegetable Stir-Fry

Ingredients:
1. 4 oz boneless, skinless chicken breast, thinly sliced
2. 1 cup mixed stir-fry vegetables (such as bell peppers, broccoli, and snap peas)
3. 1 tablespoon low-sodium soy sauce
4. 1 teaspoon sesame oil
5. 1/4 teaspoon minced garlic
6. Cooked brown rice (optional, for serving)

Preparation:
- Heat sesame oil in a skillet over medium heat.
- Add minced garlic and sliced chicken breast to the skillet and cook until chicken is cooked through.
- Add mixed stir-fry vegetables to the skillet and cook until tender-crisp.
- Stir in low-sodium soy sauce and cook for an additional minute.
- Serve over cooked brown rice if desired.

Nutritional Information (per serving, without rice):
- Sodium: 120mg
- Potassium: 250mg
- Phosphorus: 100mg
- Protein: 20g
- Calories: 220

4. Lentil and Vegetable Soup

Ingredients:
1. 1/2 cup dried green lentils, rinsed
2. 2 cups low-sodium vegetable broth
3. 1 cup diced carrots
4. 1/2 cup diced celery
5. 1/2 cup diced onions
6. 1/2 cup chopped spinach
7. 1/2 teaspoon dried thyme
8. Salt and pepper to taste (optional)

Preparation:
- In a large pot, combine dried lentils and vegetable broth.
- Bring to a boil, then reduce heat and simmer for 20-25 minutes until lentils are tender.
- Add diced carrots, celery, onions, chopped spinach, dried thyme, salt, and pepper to the pot.
- Continue to simmer for an additional 10 minutes until vegetables are cooked through.
- Serve hot as a main dish or side dish.

Nutritional Information (per serving):
- Sodium: 150mg
- Potassium: 300mg
- Phosphorus: 200mg
- Protein: 15g
- Calories: 180

5. Turkey Meatballs with Marinara Sauce

Ingredients:
1. 4 oz lean ground turkey
2. 1/4 cup whole wheat breadcrumbs
3. 1/4 cup grated Parmesan cheese (optional)
4. 1/4 teaspoon dried oregano
5. 1/4 teaspoon dried basil
6. 1 cup low-sodium marinara sauce
7. Cooked whole wheat spaghetti (optional, for serving)

Preparation:
- Preheat the oven to 375°F (190°C).
- In a bowl, combine ground turkey, whole wheat breadcrumbs, grated Parmesan cheese, dried oregano, and dried basil.
- Form the mixture into small meatballs and place on a baking sheet lined with parchment paper.
- Bake for 15-20 minutes until the meatballs are cooked through.
- Heat low-sodium marinara sauce in a saucepan over medium heat.
- Add the cooked meatballs to the marinara sauce and simmer for an additional 5 minutes.
- Serve hot over cooked whole wheat spaghetti if desired.

Nutritional Information (per serving, without spaghetti):
- Sodium: 180mg
- Potassium: 250mg

- Phosphorus: 180mg
- Protein: 20g
- Calories: 220

6. Veggie-Packed Frittata

Ingredients:
1. 2 large eggs
2. 1/4 cup diced bell peppers
3. 1/4 cup diced onions
4. 1/4 cup diced tomatoes
5. 1/4 cup chopped spinach
6. 1/4 cup shredded low-fat cheese (optional)
7. Salt and pepper to taste (optional)

Preparation:
- Preheat the oven to 350°F (175°C).
- In a bowl, whisk together eggs until well beaten.
- Stir in diced bell peppers, onions, tomatoes, chopped spinach, shredded cheese, salt, and pepper.
- Pour the egg mixture into a greased oven-safe skillet.
- Bake for 15-20 minutes until the frittata is set and lightly golden.
- Allow to cool slightly before slicing and serving.

Nutritional Information (per serving):
- Sodium: 150mg
- Potassium: 200mg
- Phosphorus: 120mg

- Protein: 12g
- Calories: 180

7. Shrimp and Vegetable Stir-Fry

Ingredients:
1. 4 oz shrimp, peeled and deveined
2. 1 cup mixed stir-fry vegetables (such as bell peppers, broccoli, and snap peas)
3. 1 tablespoon low-sodium soy sauce
4. 1 teaspoon sesame oil
5. 1/4 teaspoon minced garlic
6. Cooked brown rice (optional, for serving)

Preparation:
- Heat sesame oil in a skillet over medium heat.
- Add minced garlic and shrimp to the skillet and cook until shrimp are pink and opaque.
- Add mixed stir-fry vegetables to the skillet and cook until tender-crisp.
- Stir in low-sodium soy sauce and cook for an additional minute.
- Serve over cooked brown rice if desired.

Nutritional Information (per serving, without rice):
- Sodium: 120mg
- Potassium: 250mg
- Phosphorus: 100mg
- Protein: 20g
- Calories: 220

8. Baked Chicken Breast with Herbs

Ingredients:
1. 4 oz boneless, skinless chicken breast
2. 1/2 teaspoon dried thyme
3. 1/2 teaspoon dried rosemary
4. 1/2 teaspoon dried parsley
5. Salt and pepper to taste (optional)

Preparation:
- Preheat the oven to 375°F (190°C).
- Season the chicken breast with dried thyme, dried rosemary, dried parsley, salt, and pepper.
- Place the seasoned chicken breast on a baking sheet lined with parchment paper.
- Bake for 20-25 minutes until the chicken is cooked through and juices run clear.
- Serve hot with steamed vegetables or a side salad.

Nutritional Information (per serving):
- Sodium: 100mg
- Potassium: 300mg
- Phosphorus: 200mg
- Protein: 25g
- Calories: 250

9. Eggplant Parmesan

Ingredients:
1. 1/2 large eggplant, sliced into rounds
2. 1/4 cup whole wheat breadcrumbs
3. 2 tablespoons grated Parmesan cheese (optional)
4. 1/4 teaspoon dried oregano
5. 1/4 teaspoon dried basil
6. 1/2 cup low-sodium marinara sauce
7. 1/4 cup shredded low-fat mozzarella cheese

Preparation:
- Preheat the oven to 375°F (190°C).
- In a shallow dish, combine whole wheat breadcrumbs, grated Parmesan cheese, dried oregano, and dried basil.
- Dredge eggplant slices in the breadcrumb mixture to coat evenly.
- Place the coated eggplant slices on a baking sheet lined with parchment paper.
- Bake for 15-20 minutes until the eggplant is tender and lightly browned.
- Remove from the oven and spread low-sodium marinara sauce over each eggplant slice.
- Sprinkle shredded low-fat mozzarella cheese over the marinara sauce.
- Return to the oven and bake for an additional 5-10 minutes until the cheese is melted and bubbly.
- Serve hot as a main dish.

Nutritional Information (per serving):
- Sodium: 180mg
- Potassium: 250mg
- Phosphorus: 150mg
- Protein: 10g
- Calories: 200

10. Tofu and Vegetable Curry

Ingredients:
1. 4 oz extra-firm tofu, cubed
2. 1 cup mixed vegetables (such as bell peppers, carrots, and peas)
3. 1/2 cup light coconut milk
4. 1 tablespoon curry powder
5. 1/4 teaspoon minced garlic
6. Cooked brown rice (optional, for serving)

Preparation:
- Heat light coconut milk in a skillet over medium heat.
- Add minced garlic and cubed tofu to the skillet and cook until tofu is lightly browned.
- Stir in mixed vegetables and curry powder.
- Simmer for 10-15 minutes until vegetables are tender.
- Serve hot over cooked brown rice if desired.

Nutritional Information (per serving, without rice):
- Sodium: 120mg
- Potassium: 200mg

- Phosphorus: 100mg
- Protein: 15g
- Calories: 180

SMOOTHIES

1. Berry Blast Smoothie

Ingredients:
1. 1/2 cup mixed berries (such as strawberries, blueberries, and raspberries)
2. 1/2 ripe banana
3. 1/2 cup unsweetened almond milk
4. 1 tablespoon plain Greek yogurt (low-fat)
5. 1 tablespoon ground flaxseed (optional)

Preparation:
- Combine all ingredients in a blender.
- Blend until smooth and creamy.
- Serve immediately.

Nutritional Information (per serving):
- Sodium: 50mg
- Potassium: 180mg
- Phosphorus: 70mg
- Protein: 4g
- Calories: 120

2. Green Power Smoothie

Ingredients:
1. 1 cup spinach leaves
2. 1/2 ripe avocado
3. 1/2 cup cucumber, peeled and chopped
4. 1/2 cup unsweetened coconut water
5. 1 tablespoon fresh lemon juice
6. Ice cubes (optional)

Preparation:
- Place all ingredients in a blender.
- Blend until smooth and creamy.
- Add ice cubes if desired for a colder consistency.
- Serve immediately.

Nutritional Information (per serving):
- Sodium: 40mg
- Potassium: 300mg
- Phosphorus: 120mg
- Protein: 3g
- Calories: 130

3. Tropical Delight Smoothie

Ingredients:
1. 1/2 cup pineapple chunks
2. 1/2 ripe banana
3. 1/2 cup mango chunks
4. 1/2 cup unsweetened coconut milk
5. 1 tablespoon shredded coconut (unsweetened)

Preparation:
- Combine all ingredients in a blender.
- Blend until smooth and creamy.
- Serve immediately.

Nutritional Information (per serving):
- Sodium: 30mg
- Potassium: 280mg
- Phosphorus: 100mg
- Protein: 2g
- Calories: 140

4. Creamy Peanut Butter Banana Smoothie

Ingredients:
1. 1 ripe banana
2. 1 tablespoon natural peanut butter (unsalted)
3. 1/2 cup unsweetened almond milk
4. 1 tablespoon honey (optional)
5. Ice cubes (optional)

Preparation:
- Combine all ingredients in a blender.
- Blend until smooth and creamy.
- Add ice cubes if desired for a colder consistency.
- Serve immediately.

Nutritional Information (per serving):
- Sodium: 70mg
- Potassium: 240mg
- Phosphorus: 90mg

- Protein: 5g
- Calories: 170

5. Creamy Coconut and Berry Smoothie

Ingredients:
1. 1/2 cup mixed berries (such as strawberries, blueberries, and raspberries)
2. 1/2 ripe banana
3. 1/4 cup coconut milk (unsweetened)
4. 1/4 cup plain Greek yogurt (low-fat)
5. 1 tablespoon shredded coconut (unsweetened)

Preparation:
- Combine all ingredients in a blender.
- Blend until smooth and creamy.
- Serve immediately.

Nutritional Information (per serving):
- Sodium: 50mg
- Potassium: 200mg
- Phosphorus: 80mg
- Protein: 4g
- Calories: 150

6. Peachy Green Smoothie

Ingredients:
1. 1 cup spinach leaves
2. 1/2 cup sliced peaches (fresh or frozen)
3. 1/2 ripe banana

4. 1/2 cup unsweetened almond milk
5. 1 tablespoon ground flaxseed (optional)

Preparation:
- Combine all ingredients in a blender.
- Blend until smooth and creamy.
- Serve immediately.

Nutritional Information (per serving):
- Sodium: 50mg
- Potassium: 220mg
- Phosphorus: 90mg
- Protein: 3g
- Calories: 130

7. Mocha Almond Smoothie

Ingredients:
- 1/2 cup brewed coffee (cooled)
- 1/2 ripe banana
- 1 tablespoon unsweetened cocoa powder
- 1 tablespoon almond butter (unsalted)
- 1/2 cup unsweetened almond milk
- Ice cubes (optional)

Preparation:
- Combine all ingredients in a blender.
- Blend until smooth and creamy.
- Add ice cubes if desired for a colder consistency.
- Serve immediately.

Nutritional Information (per serving):
- Sodium: 40mg
- Potassium: 230mg
- Phosphorus: 80mg
- Protein: 3g
- Calories: 120

8. Cherry Vanilla Smoothie

Ingredients:
1. 1/2 cup pitted cherries (fresh or frozen)
2. 1/2 cup unsweetened almond milk
3. 1/4 teaspoon vanilla extract
4. 1/4 cup plain Greek yogurt (low-fat)
5. Ice cubes (optional)

Preparation:
- Combine all ingredients in a blender.
- Blend until smooth and creamy.
- Add ice cubes if desired for a colder consistency.
- Serve immediately.

Nutritional Information (per serving):
- Sodium: 40mg
- Potassium: 190mg
- Phosphorus: 80mg
- Protein: 3g
- Calories: 110

9. Pineapple Ginger Smoothie

Ingredients:
1. 1/2 cup pineapple chunks
2. 1/2 ripe banana
3. 1/2 teaspoon grated ginger
4. 1/2 cup unsweetened coconut water
5. Ice cubes (optional)

Preparation:
- Combine all ingredients in a blender.
- Blend until smooth and creamy.
- Add ice cubes if desired for a colder consistency.
- Serve immediately.

Nutritional Information (per serving):
- Sodium: 30mg
- Potassium: 230mg
- Phosphorus: 90mg
- Protein: 2g
- Calories: 120

10. Watermelon Mint Cooler Smoothie

Ingredients:
1. 1 cup cubed watermelon
2. 1/2 cup cucumber, peeled and chopped
3. 1 tablespoon fresh mint leaves
4. 1 tablespoon lime juice
5. Ice cubes (optional)

Preparation:
- Combine all ingredients in a blender.
- Blend until smooth and creamy.
- Add ice cubes if desired for a colder consistency.
- Serve immediately.

Nutritional Information (per serving):
- Sodium: 10mg
- Potassium: 180mg
- Phosphorus: 70mg
- Protein: 1g
- Calories: 80

SNACKS AND APPETIZER

1. Veggie Sticks with Hummus

Ingredients:
1. 1 medium carrot, cut into sticks
2. 1 celery stalk, cut into sticks
3. 1/2 cucumber, sliced
4. 2 tablespoons hummus (low-sodium)

Preparation:
- Arrange carrot sticks, celery sticks, and cucumber slices on a plate.
- Serve with hummus for dipping.

Nutritional Information (per serving):
- Sodium: 50mg
- Potassium: 150mg
- Phosphorus: 50mg
- Protein: 2g
- Calories: 50

2. Greek Yogurt with Berries

Ingredients:
1. 1/2 cup plain Greek yogurt (low-fat)
2. 1/4 cup mixed berries (such as strawberries, blueberries, and raspberries)
3. 1 tablespoon chopped walnuts (optional)

Preparation:
- Spoon Greek yogurt into a bowl.
- Top with mixed berries and chopped walnuts if desired.

Nutritional Information (per serving):
- Sodium: 30mg
- Potassium: 150mg
- Phosphorus: 70mg
- Protein: 8g
- Calories: 80

3. Cucumber Avocado Rolls

Ingredients:
1. 1/2 cucumber, thinly sliced lengthwise
2. 1/4 ripe avocado, mashed
3. 1 tablespoon diced red bell pepper
4. 1 tablespoon chopped fresh cilantro
5. 1 teaspoon lime juice

Preparation:
- Lay cucumber slices flat on a plate.
- Spread mashed avocado evenly on each cucumber slice.
- Sprinkle diced red bell pepper and chopped cilantro over the avocado.
- Drizzle lime juice over the top.
- Roll up each cucumber slice and secure with a toothpick if necessary.

Nutritional Information (per serving):
- Sodium: 10mg
- Potassium: 200mg
- Phosphorus: 60mg
- Protein: 2g
- Calories: 60

4. Apple Slices with Almond Butter

Ingredients:
1. 1 medium apple, sliced
2. 1 tablespoon almond butter (unsalted)

Preparation:
- Arrange apple slices on a plate.
- Serve with almond butter for dipping or spreading.

Nutritional Information (per serving):
- Sodium: 0mg
- Potassium: 150mg
- Phosphorus: 50mg
- Protein: 2g
- Calories: 70

5. Rice Cake with Cottage Cheese and Tomato

Ingredients:
1. 1 rice cake
2. 2 tablespoons low-fat cottage cheese
3. 1 slice tomato

Preparation:
- Spread low-fat cottage cheese evenly on the rice cake.
- Top with a slice of tomato.

Nutritional Information (per serving):
- Sodium: 70mg
- Potassium: 100mg
- Phosphorus: 50mg
- Protein: 3g
- Calories: 40

6. Baked Sweet Potato Chips

Ingredients:
1. 1 small sweet potato, thinly sliced
2. 1 teaspoon olive oil
3. Salt and pepper to taste (optional)

Preparation:
- Preheat the oven to 375°F (190°C).
- Toss sweet potato slices with olive oil, salt, and pepper in a bowl.

- Arrange sweet potato slices in a single layer on a baking sheet lined with parchment paper.
- Bake for 15-20 minutes until crisp and golden brown.
- Allow to cool before serving.

Nutritional Information (per serving):
- Sodium: 50mg
- Potassium: 150mg
- Phosphorus: 50mg
- Protein: 1g
- Calories: 60

7. Tuna Cucumber Bites

Ingredients:
1. 1 can tuna in water, drained
2. 1 tablespoon plain Greek yogurt (low-fat)
3. 1/4 teaspoon Dijon mustard
4. 1/4 cucumber, sliced
5. Fresh dill for garnish (optional)

Preparation:
- In a bowl, mix tuna, Greek yogurt, and Dijon mustard until well combined.
- Spoon tuna mixture onto cucumber slices.
- Garnish with fresh dill if desired.

Nutritional Information (per serving):
- Sodium: 120mg

- Potassium: 150mg
- Phosphorus: 90mg
- Protein: 10g
- Calories: 60

8. Edamame with Sea Salt

Ingredients:
- 1/2 cup edamame (cooked and shelled)
- Sea salt to taste

Preparation:
- Steam or boil edamame according to package instructions.
- Drain and sprinkle with sea salt while still warm.
- Allow to cool slightly before serving.

Nutritional Information (per serving):
- Sodium: 5mg
- Potassium: 100mg
- Phosphorus: 50mg
- Protein: 6g
- Calories: 60

9. Bell Pepper Nachos

Ingredients:
1. 1 bell pepper, sliced into rings
2. 1/4 cup black beans, rinsed and drained
3. 1/4 cup diced tomatoes
4. 1/4 cup shredded low-fat cheese

5. 1 tablespoon chopped cilantro

Preparation:
- Preheat the oven to 375°F (190°C).
- Arrange bell pepper rings on a baking sheet lined with parchment paper.
- Fill each bell pepper ring with black beans, diced tomatoes, and shredded cheese.
- Bake for 10-12 minutes until cheese is melted and bubbly.
- Sprinkle with chopped cilantro before serving.

Nutritional Information (per serving):
- Sodium: 90mg
- Potassium: 200mg
- Phosphorus: 80mg
- Protein: 5g
- Calories: 70

10. Cottage Cheese Stuffed Cherry Tomatoes

Ingredients:
1. 6 cherry tomatoes
2. 2 tablespoons low-fat cottage cheese
3. Fresh basil leaves for garnish (optional)

Preparation:
- Cut the tops off the cherry tomatoes and scoop out the seeds and pulp.
- Fill each cherry tomato with low-fat cottage cheese.
- Garnish with fresh basil leaves if desired.

Nutritional Information (per serving):
- Sodium: 50mg
- Potassium: 100mg
- Phosphorus: 50mg
- Protein: 3g
- Calories: 30

BONUS

Shopping lists

Proteins:
1. Skinless chicken breast
2. Lean ground turkey
3. Salmon fillets
4. Tofu
5. Eggs
6. Canned tuna in water
7. Low-fat cottage cheese
8. Plain Greek yogurt (low-fat)
9. Edamame
10. Hummus

Fruits:
1. Apples
2. Berries (strawberries, blueberries, raspberries)
3. Bananas
4. Oranges
5. Pineapple
6. Watermelon
7. Peaches

8. Cherries
9. Grapes
10. Lemons

Vegetables:
1. Spinach
2. Kale
3. Broccoli
4. Cauliflower
5. Carrots
6. Bell peppers (red, green, yellow)
7. Cucumbers
8. Tomatoes
9. Avocados
10. Sweet potatoes

Grains and Legumes:
1. Brown rice
2. Quinoa
3. Whole wheat pasta
4. Oats
5. Whole grain bread
6. Lentils
7. Black beans
8. Chickpeas

Dairy and Dairy Alternatives:
1. Unsweetened almond milk
2. Unsweetened coconut milk
3. Unsweetened coconut yogurt
4. Low-fat shredded cheese (mozzarella, cheddar)
5. Parmesan cheese (grated)

Nuts and Seeds:
1. Almonds
2. Walnuts
3. Chia seeds
4. Flaxseeds

Herbs and Spices:
1. Fresh basil
2. Fresh cilantro
3. Fresh mint
4. Dried oregano
5. Dried basil
6. Dried thyme
7. Dried rosemary
8. Dried parsley
9. Cumin
10. Garlic powder
11. Onion powder

Healthy Fats and Oils:
1. Olive oil
2. Avocado oil
3. Coconut oil

Condiments and Sauces:
1. Low-sodium soy sauce
2. Dijon mustard
3. Balsamic vinegar
4. Apple cider vinegar
5. Hot sauce (low-sodium)

Canned and Packaged Goods:
1. Low-sodium vegetable broth
2. Low-sodium marinara sauce
3. Unsweetened canned fruit (in water)
4. Unsweetened applesauce
5. Tomato paste (no added salt)
6. Low-sodium canned beans

Beverages:
1. Green tea
2. Herbal tea (caffeine-free)
3. Water (filtered or bottled)

Frozen Foods:
1. Frozen mixed berries
2. Frozen mango chunks
3. Frozen spinach
4. Frozen peas
5. Frozen edamame

Snacks and Appetizers:
1. Rice cakes
2. Rice crackers (low-sodium)
3. Popcorn kernels (for air-popping)
4. Low-sodium pretzels
5. Rice paper wrappers
6. Raw vegetables (carrot sticks, celery sticks, cucumber slices)

Sweeteners:
1. Honey (raw, unprocessed)
2. Maple syrup (100% pure)

Miscellaneous:
1. Unsweetened shredded coconut
2. Rice vinegar
3. Low-sodium salsa
4. Low-sodium vegetable juice
5. Low-sodium salad dressing
6. Low-sodium chicken bouillon cubes
7. Unflavored gelatin

For Breakfast:
1. Rolled oats
2. Whole grain cereal (low-sugar)
3. Ground cinnamon
4. Natural peanut butter (unsalted)
5. Whole wheat English muffins

For Lunch and Dinner:
1. Whole wheat tortillas
2. Whole wheat burger buns
3. Low-sodium canned tomatoes
4. Low-sodium chicken broth
5. Low-sodium soy milk
6. Low-sodium tomato sauce

For Side Dishes:
1. Low-sodium vegetable broth
2. Low-sodium vegetable juice
3. Low-sodium tomato sauce
4. Low-sodium canned beans

For Salad Fixings:
1. Dark leafy greens (romaine lettuce, spinach)
2. Red onions
3. Radishes
4. Beets
5. Carrots

For Dressings and Dips:
1. Low-sodium salad dressing
2. Balsamic vinegar
3. Greek yogurt (low-fat)
4. Fresh herbs (cilantro, parsley, dill)

For Baking:
1. Whole wheat flour
2. Baking powder
3. Baking soda
4. Unsweetened cocoa powder

For Cooking:
1. Cornstarch
2. Low-sodium chicken broth
3. Low-sodium vegetable broth
4. Low-sodium canned tomatoes

For Seasoning:
1. Salt substitute (potassium chloride)
2. Garlic powder
3. Onion powder
4. Paprika
5. Ground black pepper

For Beverages:

1. Green tea bags
2. Herbal tea bags (peppermint, chamomile)
3. Coffee beans (if tolerated)
4. Lemon juice

For Snacks and Desserts:
1. Unsweetened applesauce
2. Low-sugar fruit preserves
3. Dark chocolate (at least 70% cocoa)
4. Rice cakes
5. Nuts (almonds, walnuts)
6. Seeds (chia seeds, flaxseeds)

For Frozen Desserts:
1. Frozen fruit (berries, mango)
2. Unsweetened coconut milk
3. Low-sugar fruit juice
4. Unsweetened cocoa powder
5. Sugar-free gelatin

For Quick Meals:
1. Canned beans (black beans, kidney beans)
2. Canned tuna in water
3. Instant brown rice

CONCLUSION

As we reach the end of "Nourishing Wellness: A Kidney Disease Diet Cookbook for Seniors," we reflect on the journey we've embarked upon together. This cookbook was created with the utmost care and dedication, with the singular aim of supporting seniors with kidney disease in their pursuit of health, happiness, and delicious meals.

Throughout these pages, we've explored a variety of recipes carefully crafted to meet the specific dietary needs of individuals managing kidney disease. From wholesome breakfasts to hearty dinners, and delightful snacks in between, each recipe has been thoughtfully designed to be low in sodium, potassium, and phosphorus, while still providing essential nutrients and mouthwatering flavors.

But this cookbook is more than just a collection of recipes. It's a testament to the resilience and creativity of seniors facing the challenges of kidney disease. It's a resource for caregivers, family members, and healthcare professionals seeking to provide support and nourishment to their loved ones. And it's a celebration of the joy that comes from sharing nutritious, delicious meals with those we care about most.

As we bid farewell, we want to express our heartfelt gratitude to everyone who contributed to the creation of this cookbook. From the dedicated healthcare professionals who provided invaluable guidance and expertise, to the seniors who inspired us with their strength and determination, and to the caregivers and family members who offer unwavering support and love each day – thank you.

I hope that the recipes and insights shared in this cookbook will serve as a source of inspiration and empowerment for seniors with kidney disease everywhere. May each meal be a reminder of the power of nourishing both body and soul, and may each bite be savored with gratitude and joy.

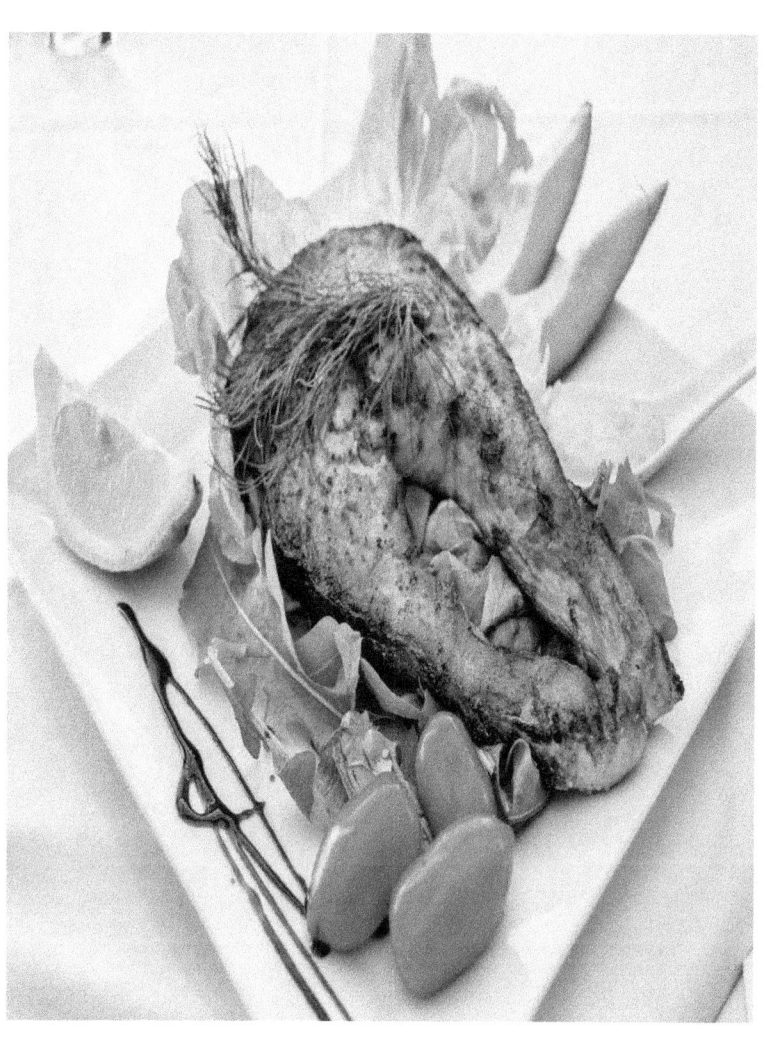

www.ingramcontent.com/pod-product-compliance
Lightning Source LLC
Chambersburg PA
CBHW070358230526
45471CB00006B/2633